Ketogenic diet

Fast weight loss tips for beginners and keto low carb recipes

Table of Contents

Introduction

I want to thank you and congratulate you for downloading the book, *"Ketogenic diet: Fast weight loss tips for beginners and keto low carb recipes"*.

This book contains proven steps and strategies on how to transform your life so that you are healthier, thinner and more energized.

You will be more enlightened about the practical steps you can employ to maximize the benefits of the ketogenic diet. This book also provides you with vital measures you should implement to avoid common mistakes.

The ketogenic diet is not about restricting your level of gratification. Instead, it is about having a tactical approach when eating the foods you love and it is our pleasure to show you how.

Thanks again for downloading this book. I hope you enjoy it!

Chapter 1: How the Ketogenic Diet Works

Foods affect your mood, weight, health and energy levels. Additionally, your body reacts differently to the amount of carbohydrates, protein and fat that you consume.

You may have constantly heard that "fat" is not good for you and instead view carbohydrates as the better option to eat. As a result, you limit your consumption of fat, but consume large proportions of carbohydrates and protein. Carbohydrates provide nutrients to the body and I'm not suggesting that they are inconsequential. However, on the ketogenic diet the amount that is eaten, should be substantially reduced.

 The body uses carbohydrates as the predominant energy source. However, there is a better and healthier alternative that the body can use. The ketogenic diet is ideal as it optimizes your body's ability to perform. The diet will make you healthier and slimmer even when exercise activity is at its lowest.

How the body functions

Foods such as grains, rice, cereals, bread, pasta, potatoes and processed sweets contain carbohydrates. During digestion, carbohydrates are further broken down into glucose which is a simple sugar. Glucose then enters the blood stream and is transported through the body to be used as energy.

When there is an excessive amount of glucose, it is stored in the muscles and liver as glycogen and it is used when blood-sugar levels are depleted. To monitor glucose levels, the body produces hormones known as insulin and glucagon.

The body's alternative

On the ketogenic diet you lower your carbs intake, consume a moderate amount of protein and high amounts of fat. Instead of carbohydrates as the energy source, fat is utilized.

So how does the body specifically utilize fat as an energy source? With a reduction of carbohydrates, less glucose enters the blood stream. In this period of adaptation the body goes through a process known as ketosis. In the state of ketosis, molecules known as ketones are created and used for energy.

Ketones are also called ketone bodies. The liver breaks down fat by first converting fat into fatty acids and the fatty acids are further broken down into ketones. The body creates three ketone bodies and they are acetone, acetoacetate and beta-hydroxybutyrate commonly abbreviated as B-OHB.

Your body's metabolism is designed in such a way that there is always an alternative when things change. It has always been that way though you may have been unaware before. With the depletion of glucose in your bloodstream, ketones are used for the body's survival. The brain can only use glucose or ketones for energy and about 20% of energy is needed for the brain.

Ketosis can take between 2-7 days to occur. In order to stay in ketosis, an individual should consume below 50 grams of net carbohydrates daily. Net carbs are total carbohydrates minus grams of fiber. So how would you know when your body is in ketosis? These are the various signs.

Signs of Ketosis

Blood Tests

There are blood sugar meters that can be used at home to test ketones or testing can be done in a lab. Blood testing gives a precise reading.

Urine

Testing your urine, is the most common way to detect ketones in the body. At the pharmacy you can obtain ketone urine-testing strips which are also known as Ketostix or ketone sticks. On the tip of these small plastic strips there is a pad made of a special chemical which changes color when ketones are in the urine. Once you abide by the directions, you will be able to determine your ketones level. On the package there are details of what the various shades of color symbolize. It is best to do this examination the first thing in the morning before eating, to obtain a more accurate reading.

You can also use the services of a health care provider to conduct the test if you do not want to do your own home test.

Variation in breath

Your normal breath may smell tangy or fruity. This is so because acetone, one of the three ketones, is purged by the body in the breath. When the body no longer has need for the extra ketones, the body does not transfer it to fat again. Instead the body eliminates it. The change in your breath is just until your body adapts. By drinking more water or chewing gum, the variation in breath can be endured without any significant discomfort during the adaptation process. Eventually, your breath will be back to normal again.

Dehydration

You may feel thirstier or your mouth may feel dry. Ensure that you drink plenty of water during this adaptation period.

Tiredness and other symptoms

You may feel tired as the body switches gears. Signs such as light-headedness, nausea and fatigue are symptoms of the process. The induction phase is also referred to as the "keto-flu". It is only for a short time and you will feel much better after a few days. Bear in mind also that you may not experience some of the keto-flu symptoms. So if you feel fine, there is no need to wonder if you are doing the diet correctly. Everyone's body reacts to diet changes differently.

Chapter 2: Advantages of the Ketogenic Diet

The ketogenic diet was originally used to treat epilepsy only, as it was discovered that during the state of ketosis, epileptic seizures were significantly diminished. Over the years, other health benefits were also discovered.

When an individual has type 2 diabetes, it means that blood glucose levels are higher than normal. The pancreas create more insulin to remedy the situation but eventually there is insulin resistance in the body. The ketogenic diet regulates the problem and reduces the need for insulin. A diabetic has to monitor his or her overall health and ensure that an unhealthy condition known as ketoacidosis does not occur. Note however, that a diabetic can use the ketogenic diet to improve his or her health.

Cancer patients also use the diet. There are studies that show that when the body is deprived of glucose, cancer cells do not thrive like before. Some individuals on the diet experienced a shrinkage of tumor growth or slowed growth. In these instances, the diet was used along with other standard cancer treatments. It all depends on how advance the cancer is. Though research is ongoing, some cancer patients have implemented the diet and have gained positive results.

Additionally, after implementing the diet, the temperament of individuals who struggle with depression or who are bipolar, improves. Individuals who are obese, find that it is easier to lose weight on the ketogenic diet than other diets.

Regardless of your health challenges, once you are on the diet, you will have more energy, think more clearly and sleep better. Your appetite will be curbed and you will have less cravings. The diet also reduces the risk of heart disease. Your blood pressure and cholesterol levels will be reduced. The body creates too much cholesterol when there is more glucose in your diet. Once your glucose levels decrease, your cholesterol levels are reduced. If you have inflammation, it will stop.

You will experience a better and more efficient thyroid performance. The thyroid gland which is in the front of your neck creates thyroid hormones. These hormones affect your breathing, metabolism, cholesterol levels, how fast or slow your brain operates, body temperature, menstrual cycles, and the heart and nervous systems. Iodine, which can be found in dairy products, salt and seafood, is needed to make the thyroid hormone.

If hormone levels are too low it is referred to as an underactive thyroid. When the glands do not produce enough thyroid hormones it is known as hypothyroidism. Symptoms include feeling cold or weary, dry skin and a slow heart rate.

When the gland produces too much hormones it is referred to as hyperthyroidism. When the gland is overactive you may feel irritable, warm or have trouble concentrating. The ketogenic diet helps to regularize hormone levels.

You will also experience better brain function and your ability to focus will improve.

Chapter 3: The Role of Exercise

Previously, you may have engaged in strenuous physical exercise but regardless of everything you've done, the weight stayed firmly in place. You may even have prolonged your exercise routine but instead of shedding pounds, you gained more weight. This is so because exercising for prolonged periods can make you so hungry that you eat more food. When you consume large amounts of carbohydrates, it usually takes about 25 minutes of exercise to burn fat. On the ketogenic diet, you do not have to be active for 25 minutes to gain results. Fat is burned whether you engage in exercise or not.

On the ketogenic diet you have to completely change your mind-set. Just as your body will be programmed differently, so too should your mind. Once your objective is to lose fat, whether it is around your waist, hips, arms or thighs, on this diet you should not include exhaustive and strenuous exercise to your routine if you have never done so before. Other than low carbs, moderate protein and high fat, the diet does not dictate that you over-exercise until you feel like collapsing. If your exercise routine is bike riding or walking, you do not need to sign up to lift heavy weights in the gym or run a marathon. If your routine is usually 40 minutes of activity, three times a week, there is no need to work out for two hours seven days a week and still worry about increasing it to three hours.

Stop worrying and allow your body to do the work for you. On the ketogenic diet, the main thing is for you to reduce your carbohydrates intake and eat more fat from the prescribed list of foods given in chapter 5. The ketogenic diet suppresses your appetite. Thus you will eat less anyway, yet still feel satiated.

In summary, you will lose weight regardless of your physical activity. Weight is lost when you eat correctly on the diet.

So what is the role of exercise? Does it mean that you should not exercise at all?

If you regularly exercise and are on the diet, it accelerates the time period in which you will lose weight. However, exercise should not be viewed as a weight loss activity only. There are many benefits when you engage in exercise. If you loathe exercise, change your way of thinking.

The Benefits of Exercise

Exercise enables your muscles to obtain oxygen and nutrients much better. Thus with a more efficient cardiovascular system you will feel supercharged and have more energy. Have you ever noted that when you are weary and it feels like you are about to fall asleep, once you become active, the feeling goes away and you feel more energized? It is because exercise increases your energy.

Moreover, when you exercise, blood and oxygen, flow better to your brain and chemicals are released causing you to concentrate better. By being more active you strengthen your heart and lower the risk of heart disease.

Exercise also maintains the flexibility of your joints, ligaments and muscles, reduce the effects of aging and improves your immune system. For diabetics, consistent exercise helps to regulate blood glucose levels.

Therefore your health will be at its optimum peak when you combine the importance of exercise and the many health benefits of the ketogenic diet.

New Exercisers

If you do not exercise and want to start, you can perform moderate intensity exercise such as brisk walking, swimming, dancing and gentle cycling. Ensure that you drink lots of water to keep you hydrated. Gradually, when your body has adapted to the diet you can progress to more vigorous exercise if you wish like fast cycling, power walking, running and aerobics.

Intense Exercisers

Individuals who engage in rigorous exercise and are new to the diet should be aware of certain factors. On the ketogenic diet you will not lose your lean muscles. Body builders use the diet yet still continue with their routine.

However, when you first start the diet, you may find it difficult when performing your vigorous exercise routines. The reason for this, is that there is an absence of glycogen in the muscles. As previously explained, when there is too much glucose, it is stored in the muscles and liver as glycogen. As carbohydrates are limited, there will be a depletion of glycogen in the muscles.

What you can take so that your regular exercise routine is not challenging, is a supplement like coconut oil before exercising to provide you with energy. This is further discussed in Chapter 5 under the heading "Dietary Tips".

There are three categories of the ketogenic diet. There is the standard ketogenic diet that is more commonly used, the cyclical ketogenic diet and targeted ketogenic diet. Thus far, we have been focusing on the standard ketogenic diet.

The cyclical ketogenic diet or the targeted ketogenic is better suited for the lifestyle of an extreme exerciser. Targeted ketogenic diet allows you to consume carbs around exercise time. Cyclical ketogenic diet allows dieters to be on the standard ketogenic diet for 5 or 6 days with a period of consuming high carbohydrates for 1 or 2 days.

Nonetheless, those options are the more advanced types of the diet and should not be implemented until you have already been on the standard ketogenic diet for at least 8-12 weeks. This is to ensure that your body first adapts to using fat for energy.

Moreover, the cyclical and targeted ketogenic diets are utilized by individuals who are already lean and who regularly engage in high-intensity exercise like body building and weight lifting. If you do not usually push your body to the limit, like weightlifters, then you should remain on the standard ketogenic diet.

Chapter 4: Ketogenic Diet Mistakes

Having the wrong perspective about the keto-flu

As previously mentioned, the body goes through a phase as it begins to use fat for energy. In this induction stage, many individuals experience flu-like symptoms such as nausea, fatigue, headaches and light-headedness. This feeling is also known as the keto-flu but it is just for a few days. The time period depends on your body's ability to adapt.

During this induction period, one major mistake many people make is to quit because of the flu-like symptoms. A few days of symptoms compared to a life time of health benefits, pale in comparison. Therefore, you should remain on your diet course.

You may have the view that the symptoms mean that your body has rejected the diet, but this is not so. When you have a cold or a flu, your immune system is usually hard at work so that you can be your normal self again. A runny nose is your body's way of expelling germs and sinuses. Muscle aches signal that your body is using protein from your muscles. You may find it annoying and feel lousy but these symptoms are just an indication that the body is expelling what is not needed and restoring itself. It is a part of the process and surely, you have survived colds and flus. Likewise, the keto-flu is a part of the process and in time the flu-like symptoms will pass. As time progresses, you won't even remember this minor hurdle, as you reap the benefits.

Consuming too many carbohydrates

For the body to go into ketosis, you must limit your carbohydrate intake to under 50 grams of net carbs per day. Many individuals consume closer to 100 grams and even 150 grams of carbohydrates which is not low enough. The body will continue to use carbs as the main source of energy instead of fat.

Eating too much protein

Additionally, consuming more protein than you need, hinders the body from entering the ketosis stage because the body converts excessive protein into glucose. Remember the objective of the ketogenic diet is to limit the amount of glucose in the body so it is not used for energy. Thus consuming too many carbs and too much protein means that you are on a different plan diet altogether.

Not eating enough healthy fat

Another mistake is reducing your carbs but not eating enough fat. Without energy being sourced from carbs or fat, it will cause the body not to properly function. There must be a balance of your nutrients on the ketogenic diet. Therefore, you must consume the right amount of healthy fat.

Confusing Ketosis with Ketoacidosis

You must frequently check your ketone level. If you are a diabetic or alcoholic this is very important. Excessive amounts of anything, can have an unfavorable impact. For example, too much sodium in the bloodstream causes high blood pressure and too much calcium in the body can cause muscle and abdominal pain. Likewise for diabetics, high blood sugar levels because of the lack of insulin, and the acidic condition that the body finds itself in, creates a condition known as ketoacidosis. In other words, insulin deficiency causes blood sugar levels to be out of control. A grave mistake that people make is to confuse ketosis and ketoacidosis. They are completely differently. Ketosis is a natural body state but ketoacidosis is a sign that the body is in an unhealthy state. Diabetics actually use the ketogenic diet for the health benefits. If you are a diabetic use the services of informed health care providers to ensure that ketoacidosis does not occur.

Bypassing the standard ketogenic diet

As a beginner, you must ensure that you commit to the standard ketogenic diet. The cyclical ketogenic diet and the targeted ketogenic diet are not for beginners. You will not reap the proper results if you bypass the standard version. The cyclical and targeted versions are utilized by people who need carbs for their workout, who are already fit and who have endured at least 8-12 weeks on the standard ketogenic diet.

Not using supplements when needed

As insulin levels decrease, and as you drink more fluids, sodium is flushed out of the body. However, the body needs sodium. Thus you need to supplement your sodium consumption by taking supplements and/or consuming foods such as chicken broth, to maintain sodium levels. If you do not supplement your diet with sodium, you may experience fatigue and dizziness. When you feel dizzy, consume more sodium, monitor how you feel thereafter and take note so you can know what to do in the future.

Not monitoring or seeking treatment for health conditions

If you are a diabetic and you're using the ketogenic diet, monitor your diabetic condition. Likewise people who suffer with their thyroid gland should also seek the proper treatment if their problems persist. One of the mistakes some people make is blaming the ketogenic diet for external health problems. If you have problems with your thyroid, it should not be assumed that the diet is at fault. Some individuals have found complete relief on the diet whereas others may need to seek treatment specifically for their thyroid gland.

Alcohol Consumption

During the early stage as your body adjusts, it is best to avoid alcohol. Later when your body has adapted to the diet, you can drink in moderation. Drinking alcohol disrupts ketosis and the body actually uses alcohol as fuel. The objective is for the body to use fat as energy and not anything else. Additionally, the hangover from alcohol coupled with the keto-flu will make you think that the diet is at fault, when in reality it is the effects of the hangover.

Intolerance

Quitting at the first sign of discomfort or because you have not lost weight instantly, is a mistake. Remember that your body is a machine, and changing your routine will cause the body to shift gears. It will take a few days for the body to adjust. Impatience and erroneously thinking that two days of reducing carbohydrates should cause you to lose twelve pounds, is being unrealistic. You will definitely lose weight but the body must first surpass the induction phase.

Chapter 5: How to Start the Diet

You must be mindful of the foods that you should and should not eat. On the ketogenic diet, you do not have to endure hunger. You can still enjoy delectable treats that will leave you full and satiated.

Foods you can eat

Fat can be categorized as good and bad. Bad or unhealthy fat induces harmful cholesterol and causes inflammation. The good type of fat promotes healthy digestion, helps the body to absorb vitamins and minerals and improves brain function. This type of fat is found in avocados, nuts, coconut oil, butter, olive oil, cod liver oil and ghee. Thus include them in your diet.

On the ketogenic diet, you should consume healthy fats, dairy products, grass fed meat such as lamb and beef, poultry, fish and seafood, pastured pork, cured and deli meats, eggs, bacon and gelatin. When purchasing fish, note that wild caught is better than farmed fish.

You can eat fruits and vegetables on the ketogenic diet but you have to know what type is best. You can eat avocado which is the main fruit and can be eaten as often as you like. These other fruits can be eaten occasionally: strawberries, blackberries, raspberries, cranberries and mulberries, honeydew melons, watermelon, cantaloupe.

Fruits that should be eaten rarely include orange, plums, apples, grapefruit, pear, kiwi and cherries. Even if you opt not to eat these fruits at all, it is okay because they should only be eaten in small amounts and not regularly as the other fruits.

On the ketogenic diet carbohydrates can be consumed. We have placed the fruits in categories so that you are aware of how often they can be eaten. Balance is key.

Other foods include vegetables such as spinach, endive, lettuce, bok choy, kale, radishes, celery stalk, asparagus, cucumber, tomato, eggplant, cabbage, broccoli, turnips, cauliflower, pumpkin and carrot. Note that some of these vegetables such as tomato, pumpkin and carrots are starchy, so you will eat them occasionally. Any vegetable or fruit that you wish to consume, you have to first determine if it is high in carbohydrates and how often you should eat it. Thus you would not eat pumpkin for breakfast, snack, lunch and dinner. You would occasionally eat it.

Also nuts such as almonds, hazel nuts, macadamia, pecans, walnuts and pine nuts, pistachio, cashew nuts can be eaten. Seeds such as sunflower seeds, flax seeds and pumpkin seeds can be consumed.

Omega-3 fatty acids is a vital part of your diet. They help to regulate your heart's rhythm, lower blood pressure, help body cells to function and generate hormones that prevent blood clotting. Sources of Omega-3 are healthy oils, mackerel, nuts dark leafy vegetables and fish such as sardines and salmon.

The body needs protein to maintain a strong immune system, muscle growth and a healthy nervous system. Sources include dairy products, fish and meat. Fiber is also important to your diet and can be obtained from leafy green vegetables and also fruit.

Flavoring and Drinks

You can use herbs, spices, lemon juice, zest, lime juice, mayonnaise, pickles, fermented foods such as sauerkraut, whey protein (without additives and artificial sweeteners), healthy zero carb sweeteners such as Stevia, cocoa powder, water, tea, coffee and coconut milk.

Ensure that you drink lots of water so that you do not get dehydrated.

Foods you should avoid eating

It is best to avoid these foods on the keto diet. Beans and legumes such as peas, kidney beans and lentils, fruit with high carbs, grains and starches such as wheat based products, bread, cereal and rice, sugary products such as sodas, ice cream and candy, artificial sweeteners such as sucralose, aspartame and cyclamates, low-fat products, potatoes, alcohol, processed vegetable oils and highly processed foods.

For every food item that you should avoid, there is a healthier substitute. If you love mash potatoes, then you will enjoy puree cauliflower. Instead of your regular bread, you can bake muffins. You can use various condiments to flavor your food and use almond flour or coconut flour, if you used a different kind before. If you wish to explore some fascinating recipes, you will be interested in our cookbook.

How to calculate your personal macros

You have to determine the macronutrients i.e. carbohydrates, proteins and fat, that you should consume for your body to be in ketosis.

A 400 lb. male and a 200 lb. female can be on the ketogenic diet for example but their macronutrients will be totally different. Therefore, each individual has to specifically determine what should be consumed daily. You cannot assume how much you should take or pattern your diet on what someone else is doing, because everyone's metabolism, overall health and exercise activity, influence the level of macros.

As a guide, the breakdown of macronutrients on the diet is 75% fat 20% protein and 5% carbohydrates. This is just a general guideline. To be more specific and to be able to determine what ratio is best for you, you have to know the amount of calories you burn daily. Your daily amount of calories is referred to as your Total Daily Energy Expenditure and is abbreviated TDEE.

At this stage to calculate your TDEE, you will need to know your weight and height. Go online and type in Keto Calculator in your search platform. Once you have opened a calculator from any website of your choice, enter your information.

For our example, we will use Sam who is 34 years old, weighs 250 pounds and is 5 feet 5 inches. Entering the information on the Keto Calculator, along with his age and gender, Sam is informed from the information that his Base Metabolic Rate is 1994 kcal. This means when he is resting and is inactive, he burns 1994 calories. Sam also wants to know his TDEE.

The next section on the Keto Calculator, has various options to select and that is whether, a person exercises, is lightly active, moderately active or very active. Sam is lightly active and selecting that option, reveals that his TDEE is 2457 calories. Do not worry about the math. The calculator works out everything for you.

The Keto Calculator also estimates that his body fat is around 41%. To obtain an accurate reading for body fat, you can purchase a body fat analyzer or measure your skin folds with skin fold calipers. Sam also has the option of measuring his hips, upper thigh and the largest part of his forearm and entering the information on a Body Fat Calculator to determine his body percentage fat. This calculator can be accessed online on various websites.

With 41% body fat, the Keto Calculator reveals that Sam has 147 lbs. of lean body mass and 102 lbs. of body fat. In order to stay in ketosis, an individual should consume below 50 grams of net carbs every day. Net carbs is calculated by subtracting grams of fiber from total carbs. Remember that everyone's body adapts to the induction phase differently. Sam decides to commit to 30 grams of net carbs daily. Note that the amount of carbs is changeable and can be tweaked according to what best works for you.

With the net carbs chosen, the Keto Calculator suggests that Sam should eat about 118 grams of protein daily. If Sam will do absolutely no exercise whatsoever, then 89 grams of protein will suffice and if he is very active 146 grams should be consumed. Using an average of the two figures (89 + 146 = 235 /2 =117.5 rounding off to nearest figure) since Sam is lightly active, Sam will consume 118 grams of protein daily.

30 grams of carbohydrates and 118 grams of protein is 592 calories according to the Keto Calculator. Sam will commit to reducing the rest of the calories by 20% so he enters this on the Calculator and becomes aware that with a

20% reduction, it means that he will consume 153 grams of fat.

Therefore to lose weight, Sam's personal macronutrients are:

1966 daily caloric consumption

30 grams of carbohydrates (6%, 120 calories)

118 grams of protein (24%, 472 calories)

153 grams of fat (70%, 1374 calories)

Sam's usual caloric intake is 2457 daily. On the ketogenic diet Sam's intake will now be 1966 daily calories which is a 20% reduction of what it was before.

Sam will be able to lose 4.1 lbs. in the upcoming days. Note that even though the calculator may project that you may lose the weight in four weeks' time, it is just a projection. You could lose that weight in a week or two. It all depends on your level of activity and other factors such as how your body adapts to the diet.

Remember also that 118 grams of protein was an average. The lowest amount of protein Sam should consume is 89 grams and the maximum is 146 grams. The calculator provides this information.

Likewise with the fat macro, the lowest amount is 30 grams and the maximum is 207 grams. Let's say that you went to dinner and consumed something that was not in your plan and when you did the calculation later, you realized that your daily consumption was 170 grams of fat instead of 153 grams. That is okay because remember that your maximum amount is 207 grams if you are very active. The following day, you will continue with your plan and continue to exercise. Do not panic and starve yourself for 24 hours to compensate for the indulgence of 17 grams (170-153) of fat.

Diet Tips

It is easy to avoid anything, once it is not in close proximity. Therefore, you should take an inventory of your pantry, cupboards and refrigerator. If you live alone, remove the foods you should not eat and give them away or when they are finished and you are ready to commit to the ketogenic diet, do not replace them. If you have a family or a housemate, separate your food. In that way you know what section of the kitchen you should rummage through to find your products.

During the induction phase you may need to take sodium, magnesium and potassium supplements.

As your body converts to the diet and sheds stored carbohydrates, your body eliminates sodium and water. Sodium helps your body to control water retention and is needed to send electrical signals so that the brain and nervous systems function well. The low energy and light-headedness that you may experience may be caused by low blood pressure and not necessarily all due to the low blood sugar. To combat this, use bouillon cubes, drink chicken broth or use electrolyte tablets. If you normally exercise and are new to the diet, ensure that you take your sodium supplement about 30 minutes before exercise.

Another supplement for when you exercise is Medium Chain Triglyceride Oil (MCT Oil) or you can use Coconut Oil. These oils improve your energy levels for your exercise routine.

Some individuals experience leg cramping and muscle unease which may be attributable to low magnesium. Therefore you can use a magnesium supplement if your body needs it. Between 300-500 mg of magnesium daily is sufficient.

Potassium helps the body to control its acid balance and is needed for the functioning of the heart and normal muscles. It can be obtained by eating foods such as yogurt, broccoli, fish and meat.

It all depends on how your body adapts. Do not take supplements in large doses because a friend does the same thing. On the ketogenic diet, you will get to know more about your body and what works best for you. Pay attention to your body and when you use supplements note the difference. If you are unsure, consult a health care provider. Simple urine and blood test can determine what nutrients are lacking and what supplements you should take.

Now that you are aware of what to eat, you can plan ahead and prepare your meals. We have included three recipes to get you started.

Chapter 6: Recipes

Ricotta and Scrambled Eggs

Serving: 1

(Calories 598, 5 grams of carbohydrates, 28 grams of protein, 45 grams of fat, 0 fiber)

Ingredients

2 whole eggs

50g Italian dry salami

1 teaspoon rosemary (fresh or dry)

150g ricotta cheese (2% fat)

salt and pepper to taste

1 tablespoon of olive oil

Directions

Slice salami into small cubes. In a small pan pour oil and fry salami cubes.

Whisk eggs and then add rosemary, salt and pepper. Include cheese in the egg mixture. Break lumps using a fork and beat mixture properly. Add mixture in the pan and cook until done.

Lemon Chicken

Servings: 3

(Per serving: 603 calories, 1.3 grams of carbohydrates, 42 grams of protein, 50 grams of fat, 0 fiber)

Ingredients

50 g. of Camembert (cheese)

salt for flavoring

1 teaspoon of ground pepper

15 olives

3/4 cup of olive oil

juice from 1 small lemon

1 tablespoon ground rosemary (or 1 cup fresh rosemary)

500 g skinless and boneless chicken breast fillets

Directions

In a medium-sized mixing bowl, mix lemon juice, some of the oil, rosemary and ground pepper. Chop chicken fillets in cubes and add it to the mixture. Let it marinade in the refrigerator for at least 2 hours. When chicken is taken out of the refrigerator, add salt.

In a non-stick frying pan, cook chicken over a medium heat until lemon juice evaporates. Pour the remainder of the oil into the pan and stir chicken until slightly brown. When ready, drain the chicken cubes and serve with olives and Camembert.

Baked Herb Salmon

(For every ½ lb. serving: 353 calories, 2 grams of carbohydrates, 32 grams of protein, 23 grams of fat, 1 gram of fiber)

Ingredients

1 teaspoon minced garlic

1 teaspoon oregano leaves

1/2 cup chopped fresh mushrooms

4 oz. butter

1/2 teaspoon ground ginger

1/2 teaspoon rosemary

1/2 cup chopped green onions

1/4 teaspoon tarragon

2 lbs. salmon fillets

4 oz. sesame oil

1/2 cup tamari soy sauce

1/2 teaspoon basil

1/4 teaspoon thyme

Directions

You have to first marinade the salmon for 1-4 hours. If the salmon is one large fillet, cut it into ½ lb. portions. Mix the sesame oil, tamari soy sauce, herbs and spices. Place the salmon into a Ziploc bag and pour the mixture in the bag. Seal the bag properly and put it in the refrigerator, ensuring that the salmon is placed skin side up.

Heat oven to 350°F. At the bottom of a large baking pan, line with foil and transfer fillet and marinade into the pan. Ensure fillet is in a single layer in the pan and bake for 10-15 minutes.

In the meantime, melt butter, then mix in the vegetables. Take salmon out of the oven and pour the vegetable mixture on each salmon fillet. Bake at the same temperature for another 10 minutes then serve.

Conclusion

Thank you again for downloading this book!

I hope this book was able to help you to become more aware of the benefits of the ketogenic as well as provide information on how the body operates.

The next step is to maintain your healthy lifestyle. Once you have attained the weight you have always dreamed of, ensure that you continue to eat correctly and exercise regularly.

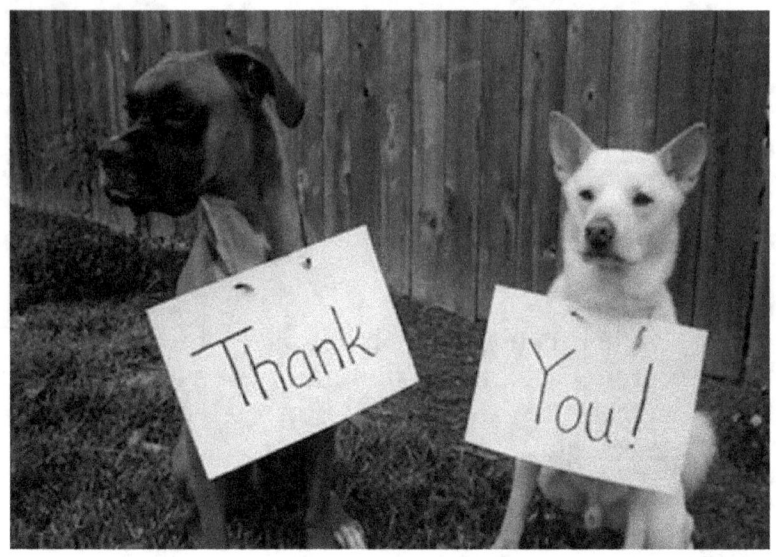

Finally, if you enjoyed this book, then I'd like to ask you for a favor, would you be kind enough to leave a review for this book on Amazon? It'd be greatly appreciated!